How to Understand and Deal with Social Anxiety

Mita Mistry

T0190781

Originally published in the UK by Vie Books, an imprint of Summersdale Publishers, part of The Octopus Publishing Group Ltd., in 2022. First published in revised form in North America by The Experiment, LLC, in 2024.

Mita Mistry has asserted her right to be identified as the author of this work in accordance with sections 77 and 78 of the Copyright, Designs and Patents Act 1988.

The Experiment, LLC
220 East 23rd Street, Suite 600
New York, NY 10010-4658
theexperimentpublishing.com

This book contains the opinions and ideas of its author. It is intended to provide helpful and informative material on the subjects addressed in the book. It is sold with the understanding that the author and publisher are not engaged in rendering medical, health, or any other kind of personal professional services in the book. The author and publisher specifically disclaim all responsibility for any liability, loss, or risk—personal or otherwise—that is incurred as a consequence, directly or indirectly, of the use and application of any of the contents of this book.

The Experiment's books are available at special discounts when purchased in bulk for premiums and sales promotions as well as for fund-raising or educational use. For details, contact us at info@theexperimentpublishing.com.

Library of Congress Cataloging-in-Publication Data available upon request

ISBN 979-8-89303-024-2
Ebook ISBN 979-8-89303-025-9

Cover and text design by Summersdale Publishers

Manufactured in the United States of America

First printing September 2024

Contents

Introduction   4

Part 1: Understanding Social Anxiety   6

Part 2: How to Manage Social Anxiety   41

Conclusion   127

Introduction

Social connection is more important now than ever. With mental health issues on the rise in an increasingly digitally engaged world, many people feel isolated, a little bit lost or afraid of what lies ahead. A recent study found social anxiety is fast-growing among young people around the world, but many do not understand the difficulties they experience in their daily functioning and well-being.

Trying to re-enter society—particularly after a period of extended isolation or self-imposed solitude—can be anxiety-inducing. The fear of social awkwardness, going back to work or relationships fizzling out can be terrifying.

Whatever you feel, it's important to understand if social anxiety might be affecting you or someone you know. This book will help you become better informed so you can learn to recognize difficulties and deal with them.

It will be helpful to have a notebook or journal on hand that you can write in during the exercises.

PART 1

Understanding Social Anxiety

Social anxiety is one of the most common types of anxiety and can affect anyone, but it's not something we talk about very much. If you suffer with social anxiety, you're certainly not alone.

The profound impact of social connection shouldn't be overlooked—it's essential to mental well-being. Anyone can learn how to lessen social anxiety and increase joy in interactions. But first, we need to understand if we have issues with social interaction. Here, you'll be guided through recognizing social anxiety: the first positive step in nurturing your mental health to becoming stronger in yourself and your connections.

What is social anxiety?

Social anxiety is an overwhelming fear of social situation, often including feeling fearful about doing something humiliating or embarrassing in front of people, and the need to come across well. Let's face it, no one likes to be judged or watched closely. It's perfectly normal for most people, even the most confident among us, to experience that feeling of dread before public speaking or to feel a little anxious before a date or meeting new people.

Social anxiety, sometimes known as social phobia, is not just about being shy or nervous. It's when intense fear or dread of social situations starts to creep into everyday life and stops us from doing the things we love.

For some people, social anxiety is limited to certain situations, like finding someone attractive or eating in public. For others, it might interfere with their functioning at work, in school and in relationships.

How does it affect you?

When we experience social anxiety, we often feel we're fundamentally flawed and not "good enough." As a result, we are extremely self-conscious about what people think of us. The fear of being humiliated triggers the "fight-flight-freeze" response, causing changes to our thoughts, bodies and behavior.

If you're struggling with social anxiety, any extra stress can make every day feel like you're swimming in an ocean with no land in sight: it can be tough. Overwhelming worry undermines your self-esteem, self-worth and confidence, leaving you feeling frustrated for not doing the stuff you love, which may lead to resentment. But it doesn't have to be this way. Anxiety is a very normal human experience: a little bit is OK and healthy to motivate you. Even though it might feel out of control or too big to manage, regaining and building confidence is entirely possible.

Who gets it?

Social anxiety is the third most common mental health issue in the world, and it often goes untreated. Anyone can worry about social situations regardless of age, gender or background.

We all have social fears, but they can vary depending on cultural customs: a form of behavior that is acceptable in one culture may not be in another. For example, a study found the fear of coming across as uninteresting in conversation triggered social anxiety among those surveyed in the West, while those surveyed in Japan said it was the fear of offending others.

Even social expectations in the same culture between different generations may vary. Younger people might scroll through their phones during meals while older people might consider it rude. It's important to understand that while social anxiety can affect anyone, a range of social rules and expectations can trigger it.

Social anxiety spectrum

Sometimes social anxiety is referred to as social awkwardness, shyness or social phobia. Although they are not entirely alike, there is overlap in how they affect our thoughts, feelings and behavior. So the same understanding and strategies can be used to help, whether the anxiety is mild, occasional or severe.

It's helpful to see the range of emotions and frequency of social anxiety to help us understand how it might be affecting us.

Occasional	Often	All the time
Social awkwardness	Shyness	Social phobia or social anxiety disorder
Discomfort in some situations	Fearful in many situations	Intense fear in most situations

All of us have experienced the fleeting embarrassment of a socially awkward situation, like waving at someone we don't know, sending a text to the wrong person or dropping items at the checkout in front of a long line. Or you might imagine climbing out of a swimming pool and your child accidentally pulling your swimsuit down in front of an audience. How awkward would that be?

Then there is shyness. Do you stick to your friend like superglue at a party, or shrink in your chair to avoid speaking up in a meeting, despite having great ideas? Everyone experiences this nervousness at some point in their lives.

Social phobia or social anxiety disorder are the next level and are very common. Often starting during teenage years, for some it gets better with age, but for others it can still creep up. It's when everyday situations stress you out, like those sleepless nights before a job interview or avoiding activities that involve seeing people face-to-face. With conscious effort it can improve, but if the distress has been present for six months or longer it is important to get help.

Which situations do you feel socially anxious in?

Most people find themselves overthinking and anxious in various situations. Here are some that can cause distress, though there are certainly more. Which situations do you find yourself overthinking? The more situations you agree with, the more socially anxious you likely are.

- Meeting new people
- Speaking with authority figures (teachers, bosses, doctors)
- Being in the limelight or center of attention
- Parties, any social gathering
- People watching me eat, drink or fill in forms
- Speaking on the phone/video call
- Being ignored in a group
- Texting or emailing someone I don't know very well
- Talking to someone I find attractive
- Returning purchases

Even if you only agree with a few situations on the list, practicing tips from this book will still help you.

Online anxiety

Of course, there are many other contexts in which you can feel socially anxious, including social media. While it's great for keeping us connected and you can control what you share, who you socialize with, mute or unfollow, many worry about being publicly judged which can make interacting online stressful. Anxious people can feel just as self-conscious online as they do in person. Imagine spending an entire day thinking about what to post online and when you do, it feels like everyone is staring at you and judging you.

Some people are anxious that a WhatsApp message might come across dull or a tweet might upset followers, which makes them hide and not share much about themselves or not take part in conversations. Video chats like FaceTime or Zoom are also problematic when people fear looking nervous or blushing online.

What's happening in your body?

When social anxiety strikes, you may experience physical reactions. Even the thought of meeting new people, attending an event or speaking in front of a group can trigger changes in your body.

Do any of these symptoms sound familiar in response to social situations?

- Racing heart or palpitations
- Shaking or trembling
- Sweating
- A choking feeling
- Shortness of breath
- Tightness in your chest
- Feeling nauseated or upset stomach
- Feeling dizzy or lightheaded
- Numbness, tingling or muscles tensing
- Blushing
- Dry throat and mouth
- Lump in throat
- Trembling voice
- Headache
- Blurred vision
- Hot flashes or chilling feeling

What's happening to your thoughts?

It's not just unpleasant physical symptoms that we experience; unhelpful thoughts can also make these dreaded situations even worse. Do you worry about what people think, or that you will say something embarrassing in front of others?

Perhaps you want to do the right "socially acceptable" thing, or you want people to like you and worry that you'll "get it wrong." Maybe you think "I'm bad at making conversation."

You might fixate on other people's reactions and worry about how you look to them or you try to guess what they think about you. Often, social anxiety sufferers assume people are judging them negatively—even more so in situations where there is a risk of being embarrassed or criticized. But negative thoughts about social situations reflect the anxiety rather than reality.

Unhelpful thoughts

We think up to 70,000 automatic thoughts a day, which is marvellous, because it shows the brilliance of our brains: we don't have to remember to get out of bed, brush our teeth, put our shoes on, walk to the store and so on.

Studies show that the majority of our automatic thoughts are negative (we all have them, it's perfectly normal and they are intended to keep us safe) but social anxiety is related to increased negative thinking. Negative automatic thoughts convince you something awful will happen, making social anxiety worse. Imagine walking into a room full of people. A negative automatic thought might pop up such as: "Everyone will think I'm odd" or "No one will talk to me."

Once you get caught up in negative thoughts, it's hard to stop them from spiralling out of control. These thoughts plant seeds of doubt which keep growing every time you give them attention; and sadly, they influence how you feel and how you behave.

While it might seem a little strange to do, it's helpful to get to know your thoughts. Whether they are about the past, present or future, socially anxious thoughts might sound like this: *I might forget what to say. I might say something embarrassing. Everyone can see me blushing. I can't stop cringing and thinking about the event afterward. I will say something stupid. They're all talking about me. My voice sounds shaky. I don't know what to say. They will think badly of me. Everyone is watching me closely. I'm so incompetent, everyone else is confident. I can't cope talking in front of a group, my words will come out wrong.*

Do any of these thoughts sound familiar? Don't worry if they do. Read on to see how to deal with them.

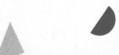

What's happening to your behavior?

You may have been at family gatherings, work events or parties where you've wanted to hide in another room, away from everyone. Perhaps you've stumbled upon a pet at a party and stayed with it to avoid people. Maybe you find excuses to avoid social situations in the first place. Or if you do go, you plan what you will say and how you will escape early. If this sounds familiar, it's quite a normal part of social anxiety.

Whichever situations you feel anxious in, not taking part in social activities (avoidance) or engaging in social activities but relying on props to make you feel comfortable—like sticking to your BFF or stroking the cat (safety behaviors)—are unhelpful and make social anxiety worse.

Loneliness

Perhaps the loneliest feeling in the world is not being understood by anyone. You might be surrounded by people but if connection is blocked by anxiety, it's hard to share your thoughts and feelings, keeping you isolated. Loneliness shames you, tricking you into believing you're invisible and don't belong; that you're not enough and it's unsafe to be yourself.

As humans, we're biologically wired for social connection to survive. So, when we're lonely, we experience it as a physical state of emergency. Imagine living in a tribe and while you're out hunting you end up alone. Without group protection, you'd feel threatened and your stress response would kick in. We still carry this instinct.

Loneliness harms our health—it's linked to dementia, Alzheimer's and depression. It deprives you of opportunities, joy and self-esteem. We all feel lonely at times, it's a normal human emotion and a sign we need more connection.

What causes social anxiety?

Social anxiety can run in families but it's unclear if it is learned behavior or genetics. Studies show that people with social anxiety have an overactive amygdala, the fear center in the brain, which elevates anxiety in social situations.

You might have learned to fear judgment through stressful and shaming childhood experiences such as criticism, bullying or being harshly judged. Fear makes you hide parts of yourself because you think you're not good enough and will be humiliated or rejected.

That fear is so real it damages your self-esteem and confidence, leaving you feeling isolated or depressed. It becomes harder to be your natural lovable self and to build meaningful connections. To others, you might seem distant, stuck-up or unfriendly when really, you're just afraid.

Social anxiety can exist alongside depression, general anxiety or autism. Please speak with your doctor if you're concerned about any aspect of your mental well-being.

What are we so afraid of?

Ultimately, we're hardwired for connection to survive and thrive, but we are afraid of people rejecting us. You worry your social skills aren't up to scratch and people will judge you for your perceived flaws.

Perhaps you worry your appearance isn't good enough because your teeth aren't straight, or you've got blemishes, and everyone will think you are unattractive, or your clothes aren't trendy enough. Maybe you're afraid of people noticing anxiety when you blush or sweat under pressure, which makes you want to crawl under a rock and disappear.

You might think your personality isn't bubbly, funny, intelligent or interesting enough and you believe you're inadequate, uncool or don't belong.

If any of this sounds familiar, you're certainly not alone. You don't need all the answers to what causes social anxiety to deal with it, but it's essential to understand what keeps it going to help break the cycle.

What keeps it going?

Imagine you're about to present to a group of people and your worst fear is your mind will go blank, you'll blush, look nervous during the presentation and will be humiliated by your colleagues. Your stress response (fight-flight-freeze) is likely to be triggered by these thoughts because they are perceived as a threat by your brain. This is the body's protective response to a threat of being attacked. When your stress response is activated, physical changes happen in your body such as your mind going blank, sweating, blushing, a racing heart, feeling sick or having panic attacks, and the anxiety itself causes the scenario you've been worrying about. It's a vicious cycle.

But often, the chances of social threat happening are overestimated by your brain (worst fears rarely happen) so it's important to be mindful of this.

What are your worst social fears?

Your beliefs also keep social anxiety going. If you've been shy or socially anxious for many years you may have developed beliefs such as "I'm not good in social situations." You might believe that "others are judgmental" or "I am not good enough" because you've been criticized for being "too quiet" or you believe "showing emotions is weak" if you've been teased for being sensitive.

If you've been bullied, you may believe "I'm unlikeable" or "I need to be popular to prove myself." If you've been held to high expectations you may believe "people will not respect me if I make a mistake" or "if people see the real me, they won't like me."

You might believe your "inferiority" is visible to others to be criticized. Unhelpful beliefs are like demons that haunt you, dragging your thoughts and self-esteem on a downward spiral—but it is possible to change them.

Take a moment to write down some of your beliefs.

Negative thoughts

As you know, negative thoughts are normal and happen automatically, planting seeds of doubt in your mind. Giving them attention keeps social anxiety growing while belittling your self-esteem, self-worth and confidence.

Negative thoughts can be words or images. You might think you will come across as boring at a party or visualize a social situation playing out like a horror film with a disastrous ending.

Consider the diagram and take a moment to write down some negative thoughts or images you have about social situations.

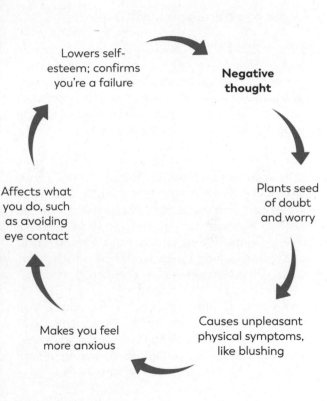

Negative
thought

Plants seed
of doubt
and worry

Causes unpleasant
physical symptoms,
like blushing

Makes you feel
more anxious

Affects what
you do, such
as avoiding
eye contact

Lowers self-
esteem; confirms
you're a failure

How you think you look to others

How do you think other people see you when you're feeling socially anxious? Imagine you are in a meeting: you're nervous and convinced everyone is staring at a sweat patch under your armpit; they can see your hands trembling and your cheeks blushing bright red.

But what you think people see and what they truly see are two different things. Perhaps they did notice the sweat patch while you were presenting and thought "It's hot in here, I should open a window" or "Ah, that can't be nice for them." Consider that people have empathy and don't always judge negatively. Even if they do, it's a poor reflection of their character!

The point is, although you feel anxious, you actually come across much better than you realize. Try this: Look in the mirror—can you see your thoughts, feelings, heart racing, palms sweating? No? Neither can other people.

Self-focused attention

Imagine having a conversation with a colleague. Your attention is entirely focused on spotting danger or questioning if you sound interesting, how you're being judged, whether the cheerful person across the room who glanced in your direction was laughing at you, what you should say next, can they see your blemishes and so on. Does it leave very much of your attention to focus on connecting with the other person, and making conversation?

It's impossible to fully listen to what people are saying or engage in meaningful chat with all those annoying thoughts racing around your mind. Self-focused attention amplifies feeling self-conscious, further preventing connections from forming or conversations flowing naturally. You also miss the chance to see how the person you are with is responding, which more often than not, is positive.

When you feel socially anxious, where is your attention focused?

Avoidance

Of course, it makes sense for us to avoid anxious situations because when we do, our worst-case scenario can't possibly come true, and we save ourselves a whole lot of distress. Sure, avoiding situations will give you some relief, but it's only temporary because your underlying idea of what is socially threatening isn't challenged or changed.

So, your social fears continue. In fact, avoidance encourages anxiety to spread to more and more situations as you start to believe that you simply can't cope with interactions. When other areas of your life such as work and relationships are affected (remember loneliness is a sign we need more connection, not to avoid it) it starts to feel bigger and bigger. That's why it's really important to understand avoidance because it keeps social anxiety going.

Which social situations do you avoid?

Safety behaviors

Imagine attending a party (fantastic, you haven't avoided a social situation) but you only talk to your best friend (safety behavior), in order to avoid your fears coming true (that everyone will judge you as boring and unattractive). Staying with your friend helps you feel more comfortable, but you've avoided challenging your fears (coming across as boring and unattractive).

Imagine having a glass of wine or two (safety behavior) then feeling bold enough to speak with someone new. Afterward, you worry all night if they thought you were wildly boring or noticed your blemishes. Despite warm conversation flowing naturally, including a compliment about your hair, you put it down to the wine (safety behavior) rather than realizing that the situation was safe, you're socially capable and this person likes your appearance.

Notice how, even though your social fears are proven wrong, your inner critic still manages to dismiss your accomplishment of meeting someone new and berates you for not hitting the mark.

Safety behaviors can look like this:

- Avoiding eye contact
- Not speaking up during discussions or meetings
- Wearing clothes that blend in to keep the spotlight away
- Asking a lot of questions, so you don't have to share personal details
- Over-preparation for presentations or meetings in a perfectionist way
- Making excuses to leave early
- Using alcohol or drugs
- Covering up your anxiety symptoms in some way, such as using makeup to cover blushing
- Having anxiety medications to hand "in case it's needed"
- Only talking to people who are "safe"
- Using headphones or hiding behind a device to avoid people striking up a conversation

You might feel like these safety behaviors help to ease anxiety and prevent your worst fears happening, but they stop you from learning that your worst-case scenario isn't true or is unlikely to happen.

What safety behaviors do you use?

Inner critic's postmortem

After a social situation, do you look back and conduct a postmortem analysis of everything that happened? Perhaps you nitpick every little detail? Then beat yourself up for all the things that you "could have" or "should have" done? Your inner critic might be shouting, "You looked ridiculous wearing jeans, you should have worn slacks like everyone else." Or, "Everyone thought you were awkwardly quiet." And, "Those jokes you made to cover up your nerves sounded cringey."

You're convinced everyone thinks like your inner critic, so it's no surprise you're anxious. But your inner critic's harsh judgments are unlikely to be 100 percent accurate. Interestingly, research shows that a socially anxious person has equal social skills to everyone else, they just don't believe it. So, isn't it about time to quiet your inner critic? You are far better than you realize—honestly, you truly are.

Shame

Our inner critic is anxiety-provoking and shaming. Shame is feeling that something about us is so terribly flawed, we don't deserve connections. Everyone experiences shame. It's almost impossible to go through life without being shamed. Whether it happens in childhood or as an adult, the outcome is the same: if no one validates you repeatedly, you learn to believe you're not worthy.

Shame makes us crawl into ourselves and keep everyone out, which triggers more avoidance behaviors to self-soothe. Shame is a big deal: it disconnects us from people, it teaches us to feel alone. It attacks our capacity to love each other and ourselves. But humans are social beings, we're hardwired for connection, love and support to survive and thrive.

Sometimes feeling shame is so vague, it's normal to be unaware of what's causing discomfort. Learning to recognize and soothe yourself through shame will help to ease social anxiety.

Pandemic trauma

It's important to understand that the coronavirus pandemic was a form of trauma on the fabric of society, leaving a devastating effect on the health and welfare of many. Let's be honest, no one is immune to the fear, isolation or anxiety caused by a crisis. For many, old childhood traumas have been re-triggered, for others it's heightened anxiety or brought it on for the first time.

In a survey by the Centers for Disease Control and Prevention, 63 percent of 18- to 24-year-olds reported symptoms of anxiety or depression. Pandemic trauma can impact brain development and increase the risk of long-term mental and physical health issues in young children whose brains and bodies are still developing.

So, our collective mental health—including social anxiety—needs greater awareness. By building social bonds that humans need to feel safe and connected, it's possible for all to recover.

Putting it all together

Social anxiety is a chain of events that might look this this:

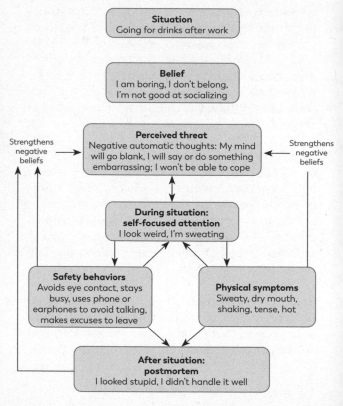

Situation
Going for drinks after work

Belief
I am boring, I don't belong, I'm not good at socializing

Strengthens negative beliefs →

← Strengthens negative beliefs

Perceived threat
Negative automatic thoughts: My mind will go blank, I will say or do something embarrassing; I won't be able to cope

During situation: self-focused attention
I look weird, I'm sweating

Safety behaviors
Avoids eye contact, stays busy, uses phone or earphones to avoid talking, makes excuses to leave

Physical symptoms
Sweaty, dry mouth, shaking, tense, hot

After situation: postmortem
I looked stupid, I didn't handle it well

Gifts of being socially anxious

Being socially anxious is not all gloom. Socially anxious people have remarkable gifts which they often don't see, and these gifts are needed in this world now more than ever.

Just take in these admirable qualities: people who struggle with small talk are often great at deep diving into topics they're passionate about. They're empathetic, helpful and considerate of other people's feelings, which makes them great listeners while being respectful of others. Such people are brilliant at building bridges, and they make great partners and the best types of friends. Everyone loves genuine people!

Consider this: because you think before speaking or sending messages, your thoughtful words lead to good first impressions and better relationships. Your built-in warning system makes you better at responding to threat. Which of course spurs your attention to detail, leading to high intelligence, achievement and creating outstanding work fuelled by high standards. Pretty amazing!

Nothing about any of us is all good or all bad. If you struggle with social anxiety, remember it's helped to shape who you are and who you are becoming in positive, healthy ways. Perhaps you're the caring friend, the attentive partner, the hardworking colleague, the empathetic leader or thoughtful sibling. Anxiety doesn't define you, it's just something that happens— and it happens to many. It's a normal part of being human that is sometimes beautiful and at other times a little messy, and that's OK. Embrace your humanity.

It may sound daunting or unbelievable, but no matter how hard it seems you can deal with social anxiety. It is entirely possible to take action and work with your strengths to change the story.

What are your strengths? (Yes, you do have them!)

Understand your social anxiety

You may already have an idea of the nature of your social anxiety by now. Some of the causes can be identified through a bit of investigation. Consider this diagram—take some time to reflect and answer the questions.

What do I believe about me?

What are my negative automatic thoughts?

What are my physical symptoms?

Self-focus: What negative images do I have of myself?

What are my avoidance or safety behaviors?

What negative thoughts happen after social events?

Journaling

It's helpful to keep a journal at any stage of reflection to deepen your understanding of yourself and deal with difficulties. Imagine yourself as a detective who is investigating a mystery. Keep an open mind. Stay curious. Write when and where you felt anxious and what was happening at that time. Make notes on your thoughts, feelings, safety behaviors and physical symptoms before, during and after the situation. There is no right or wrong way to journal. Simply write how you feel—or draw pictures if you prefer.

When everything is laid out clearly on paper it can help you to spot what is worrying you and identify patterns to work through difficulties. We might bottle up feelings because we don't want to burden others but dedicating 10 minutes each day to writing in a journal is a simple yet powerful way of empowering change and monitoring your progress.

You are not alone

Please remember social anxiety affects more people than you might realize; you're certainly not alone. Over the past few years, celebrities such as Kim Basinger, Naomi Osaka, Barbra Streisand, Donny Osmond and Adele have opened up about their struggles with social anxiety and other mental health challenges.

It can be hard to imagine that someone who comes across so confidently under the media spotlight might experience anxiety in social situations, but it happens. It's fabulous that they are speaking about it, as it's helping to open up difficult conversations and hopefully ending the stigma around social anxiety. They are living proof that you can live your life and do the things you love in the face of anxiety.

In your notebook, write a few names of people who have overcome adversity. Use this to remind yourself that you are not alone, and you certainly don't have to suffer in silence.

Hope

Hope and fear cannot occupy the same space. Invite one to stay.—Maya Angelou

Perhaps you've lost hope in your ability to change your situation. When hope is lost, you lose motivation to change. What's the point in meeting people? You're convinced you'll be rejected. What's the point in exercising? It won't make a difference.

Anxiety keeps you sinking into a miserable rut, but so many people have overcome extraordinary adversity. Reading their stories, surrounding yourself with nurturing people or joining a support network helps to build hope.

When you feel there's no light at the end of the tunnel, even taking one small step plants a seed of hope to break that helpless feeling and move forward: breathe (page 74), eat well, *tell someone*. Keep repeating and build on your progress; it makes a difference over time.

What seed of hope might you plant today?

PART 2

How to Manage Social Anxiety

Throughout the following pages, you will find a series of tips that are designed to help improve your social anxiety and leave you feeling calmer and more in control—before, during and after social situations. With tips ranging from cognitive behavioral therapy tools, mindfulness to self-care, as well as simple ideas that take a few seconds and those that require a bit more time, you will find something to help you. By taking these proactive steps toward nourishing your mental health, you are on your way to becoming better and happier in social situations and building great connections along the way.

Break the cycle

As you've seen, social anxiety can easily spiral out of control, leaving you feeling low and exhausted. But the cycle can be broken by learning ways to help yourself deal with what keeps it going. Understanding is the key—and you've already taken superb steps.

To break the cycle, it helps to:

- Change negative thought patterns and beliefs.
- Reduce self-focused attention by paying better attention to people and your environment. This builds a more accurate picture, plus it makes you less self-conscious.
- Change avoidance and safety behaviors. This requires doing things in a new way, which might seem a little scary, but it's utterly essential to break old patterns.
- Deal with the physical symptoms of anxiety, to feel more relaxed and confident in social situations.
- Face your fears: uncertainty can trigger social anxiety, so facing some fears is a game-changer.
- Practice self-care, in order to promote confidence and self-worth.

Deal with it

You don't need special skills to deal with social anxiety, but you do need to take action. It's super valuable to learn about the vicious cycle that keeps your social anxiety going, because then you can tackle breaking it. Let go of unrealistic expectations—if changes don't happen quickly, that's OK. Don't lose hope. Keep going, they will happen. Give yourself as much time as you need; and as best as you can, be kind to yourself.

Celebrate progress on good and bad days (we all have them) and don't let setbacks take over your life. Every day is a fresh new start and an opportunity to try again. Initially, if you struggle with doing things differently, that's normal. Start with easy tips first and work toward more challenging ones as your confidence grows. You've got this!

Thoughts are not facts

Our thoughts are powerful. Often at the root of many issues, they directly influence how we feel and behave more than we might realize. We've all experienced uncomfortable feelings when we've jumped to conclusions without knowing all the facts, like that time you thought your best friend was upset with you for not replying to a text, but they were actually incredibly busy. Unhelpful thoughts and thinking errors can lead us to feel truly awful.

Thoughts are not facts, and they are certainly not 100 percent accurate all of the time. It's worth remembering that people with social anxiety overestimate the chances of terrible things happening if their worst-case scenarios or social fears were to come true.

So, when a pesky thought pops up, such as "You'll always be an anxious wreck," remind yourself it's just an annoying fuzzy sound and tell it, "Nice try, you're not a fact!"

Identify negative thoughts

To challenge negative thoughts, we must first identify them. Let's get curious and investigate. Think back to a specific situation when you felt anxious. If you can't recall one, write it down the next time it happens. It might seem a little strange, or like hard work, but psychologists and therapists recommend that you get to know your thoughts: it will really help you. You might wish to write it like this:

What situation makes you anxious?	What are your feelings?	What are your thoughts?
Manager wants to talk to me	Worried, nervous	They are going to fire me
Going out to a bar	Heart racing, trembling	I don't mix in well
Friend is ignoring me	Rejected, sad, alone	I feel invisible
Saying the wrong thing	Fearful, embarrassed	I can't say anything right
Alone with an attractive person	Flustered, worried	I'm not good enough

Unhelpful thinking errors

We all make unhelpful thinking errors that cause terrible feelings. Ask yourself:

Are you taking things **personally**? "He turned away, so he's bored of me." "She looks angry probably because she's working with me."

Are you **jumping to conclusions, mind-reading or predicting the future**? "They won't invite me, they think I'm too quiet." "I'll always be a loner."

Are you **catastrophizing**? "If something goes wrong, it will be a disaster." "I will never be able to show my face at work if it goes badly."

Are you **rejecting positives**? "Thanks for the compliment, it wasn't my best work." "I'm not special."

Are you **over-generalizing**? "I'm always late." "I always forget names." "It always ends in tears."

Are you **labelling**? "I'm an idiot." "I can't even hold a conversation."

Are you **magnifying**? "Everyone is so confident and I'm not." "I messed up in a big way."

Create balanced thoughts

Balanced helpful thoughts are the kind reassuring friend we all need: the kind who is gentle yet gives you a well-rounded perspective. When our thoughts are gentle and realistic as opposed to fear-based worst-case scenarios, we're more likely to feel safe enough to open up and connect with others.

To create balanced, helpful thoughts, you must notice negative ones as soon as they pop up and get better at challenging them before they drag you down. Fight back by imagining your best friend is having these negative thoughts; what would you tell them?

Ask yourself:

- "Would I be thinking differently if I was feeling more positive?"
- "Am I considering all relevant facts about this situation?"
- "Is there any real evidence?"
- "Am I dismissing my strengths?"
- "What's the worst that could happen? Would life still go on?"
- "What's the best that could happen?"

Balanced helpful thoughts are a game-changer for social anxiety.

Helpful thinking

Now you're aware of your negative thoughts and unhelpful thinking styles, and how to challenge them, to keep them away write down as many balanced thoughts as you can. Here are some examples to get you started.

Common thinking errors	Negative thoughts	Balanced thoughts
Personalizing	They're all looking at me.	They might like my outfit.
	They must be talking about me.	Perhaps they're curious who I am.
Jumping to conclusions	She thinks I'm boring.	Maybe I can't tell what she thinks.
	He doesn't like me.	Perhaps he is as shy as I am.

Common thinking errors	Negative thoughts	Balanced thoughts
Predicting the future	I will not enjoy myself.	It could be fun.
	Everyone will think I'm odd.	People are not judging me or on a witch hunt.
Catastrophizing	If I don't present well, I'll get fired.	I'm as good as everyone else.
Rejecting positives	I just talked nonsense.	People talked to me; they do like me.

Mindfulness of thoughts

One way to stop unhelpful thoughts from wreaking havoc is the use of mindfulness, which is like pressing pause on the negative stories our thoughts tell us. By shining a light on these, we give them less power. We step back from worst-case scenarios to take a more considered perspective. Since we develop more self-awareness in the process, we're also less prone to being triggered by worry.

An excellent way to acknowledge thinking errors is to notice them like you're watching a film in your mind. The idea is to sit and watch, even though you might feel like pressing mute, stopping or fast-forwarding the film. By watching, you learn to get more comfortable with bombarding uncomfortable thoughts while training your mind to be calmer. Over time, you're barely shaken by them. Amazing!

Try this exercise for 5 to 10 minutes as best as you can. There is no right or wrong outcome, just allow your experience to be.

Close your eyes and imagine a gorgeous, calm-flowing stream. Water is gently trickling downhill over rocks and around trees. It's a beautiful day. The sun's rays warm your face and there's a gentle breeze. Every now and then a leaf falls into the water floating downstream. Imagine you are sitting on the bank watching the leaves floating by.

Every time a thought pops up, imagine it's written on one of those leaves. Stay here and let the thought leaves float by without trying to make the stream flow faster or slower. Notice whatever thoughts or feelings show up and let it be.

Practice this as many times as you can, preferably daily. Each time you notice your thoughts, you're retraining your brain to break the anxiety cycle.

Distracting negative thoughts

As you have seen, focusing on threatening thoughts before, during or after a social situation magnifies anxiety. Studies show that distractions from negative thoughts help to break the vicious cycle and stop them causing overwhelm. When we shift our attention away from upsetting thoughts and unpleasant physical symptoms, we will find they often disappear. Try these quick and easy ways to distract your attention, especially when you feel swamped:

- Count all even numbers backward from 100.
- Recite the alphabet.
- Count all the blue cars on the road.
- Guess where the people around you live.
- Think of foods you like that begin with the letter C.
- Set a worry time: only allow yourself 30 minutes a day to let bothersome thoughts run wild.

Make your own list of go-to distraction tools.

Core beliefs

Our core beliefs are deeply held assumptions about ourselves, the world and other people. Shaped by our childhood, they determine our reality and behavior. Often they're untrue, but like a magnet our attention is drawn to evidence that backs them up. They're usually the root cause of many of our issues, including our automatic negative thoughts.

Inflexible assumptions such as "I am unlovable," "People are judgmental" and "The world is unsafe" make it difficult to have balanced thoughts. You might believe you are a failure and therefore unworthy of good things, or that you're a terrible person for making a mistake and so you carry the heavy burden of shame.

If our core beliefs are positive and helpful, we're likely to be confident and happy. If they are not, our self-esteem may suffer. Because core beliefs are deeply rooted, they can be difficult to change. But the good news is, it's possible.

Uncover core beliefs

One way to uncover your core beliefs is to look for patterns in your thinking when you challenge your thoughts. You may notice common themes on what you think about yourself (I am), other people (People are) and the world (The world is).

Imagine you think "No one likes me":

"If no one likes me, it means there's something wrong with me which means I am flawed, which means I'll never be as good as others which means I am the worst. If I'm the worst, it means I'm worthless. My core belief is I'm worthless. And that feels like a slap in the face."

Your core beliefs to work on are hidden within your negative thinking patterns. Make it a habit to notice and write in your journal, like this:

I am . . .	People are . . .	The world is . . .	Themes
No one likes me.	People are judgmental.	The world is hostile.	I'm worthless.

Shift your perspective

Once you've uncovered one or more beliefs, you can challenge them. An effective way is to shift your perspective on core beliefs. Let's play devil's advocate by asking these questions:

- Is this belief in my best interest?
- Is this belief really true and valid?
- Would my younger self think it's strange that my worth is defined by others?
- Would my older self care what others think?

Consider from an alternative perspective: What might a healthier core belief be?

Consider the opposite belief might be true. Try reversing "I must hide how I feel" to saying "It's OK to show my true feelings," or "I must not get this wrong" to "It's OK and human to make mistakes." Is the reverse more true or helpful?

The point here is to show you that new beliefs are entirely possible, and how changeable (and therefore not factual) they really are.

Challenge core beliefs

Our brains love evidence, so an important way to challenge a core belief is by finding and recording proof that the belief is not entirely true. Ask yourself: "What experiences do I have which show this belief is not entirely true 100 percent of the time?"

In your journal, list as many experiences as you can remember from when you were a child to today. Even if you're unsure whether it's relevant, every small experience counts. Evidence that goes against a core belief such as "I'm a failure" or "I'm boring" could be "I passed my driving test and school exams" and "I go out with friends and receive invites to drinks with colleagues."

Challenge yourself: If you think you are worthless, boring, socially incompetent, a failure or unlovable, find three pieces of proof for each that you are not.

At this point, you might find it helpful to pay attention to what triggers unhelpful beliefs. Think back to a time when you felt ashamed or judged. How did you feel? Where were you? What were you doing? Why did you feel like you weren't enough? Who were you with when this belief surfaced? What were the triggers of your negative self-talk? Write down as much as you can. Expressing it helps to process your feelings and notice patterns.

Because core beliefs are often longstanding or emotionally charged, challenging them might feel a little hard, and that's perfectly normal. So please don't worry if you struggle with this tip, just congratulate yourself for trying. It's not an easy one, and if you find it is too tough but would like to work through it, please seek help from a mental health professional who will be able to help. You're doing amazingly, learning and changing. Keep going!

New core beliefs

New positive core beliefs happen when your behavior changes in line with them. Living with and acting on our new beliefs not only makes them stronger, it's also a super powerful way to transform old beliefs. Now is your time to create positive new beliefs and act on them. Make an action plan like this. You can do it . . . exciting times are ahead!

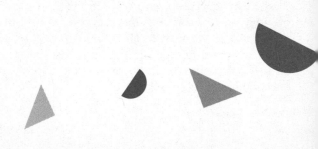

New core belief	Action	When?	Action to overcome challenges
Self: likeable Others: friendly World: safe	Contact a friend who I haven't seen for a long time to meet for coffee.	Today, to meet next week.	If they don't respond, they might be busy. Try again in two days.
Self: capable Others: supportive World: opportunities	Ask to work on a new project at work.	Speak to boss tomorrow.	If boss is busy, arrange a convenient time. If they say no to request, ask why and for alternative new opportunities.

Reduce self-focused attention

Research shows that people with social anxiety have heightened self-focus, which often leads to magnifying the worst-case scenario, second-guessing how others perceive them and misreading social situations.

You know that horrible feeling when you're convinced everyone is staring at your dishevelled hair or you think they're laughing at your socks; you've clumsily spilled a drink and now you dare not speak because your mouth is dry, and your voice will sound shaky. It's not a pleasant feeling. But fear not, it is possible to change.

Reducing self-focused attention requires you to do a little bit of attention training, which is a way of becoming aware of where your attention is focused and gaining the ability to refocus it to where you want. It's a bit like a spotlight: you can either choose to focus it on troublesome thoughts or turn it outside to focus on a person or a conversation.

Attention training

Paying attention to your senses—touch, smell, sight, hearing and taste—can literally get your attention out of your racing thoughts and into the world around you.

The idea is to use everyday activities to practice focusing your attention on a task, so when you're in a social situation, you are able to focus on the task of socializing rather than focusing on your worries. This can dramatically transform conversations and strengthen connections.

Start by noticing your breathing or sensations in the soles of your feet when you walk. Notice the smell of food before eating. Notice the sensations of water flowing on your body during a shower. Notice the smell and taste of toothpaste when brushing your teeth. If your mind wanders that's OK, simply guide it back to the task.

Practice attention training in everyday activities a few times a day.

Attention-training prompts

The beauty of attention training is you don't have to add extra stuff to your to-do list, you're simply changing how you pay attention. What everyday activities (like washing dishes, commuting, eating, getting dressed or making a cup of coffee) could you use for attention training?

Use these prompts to help you during attention training:

- Touch—where on your body do you have contact with the task? Is the texture rough or smooth, hot or cold?
- Smell—what aromas can you smell? How many are there? Are they light or heavy?
- Sight—what do you see? What are the colors, shadows, shapes or lighting?
- Hearing—what sounds can you hear? Are they loud or soft, near or far?
- Taste—what flavors do you notice? How many are there? Are any overpowering?

Focus during social situations

Once you've got attention training under your belt, you're more than ready to use this new-found skill while socializing. So, let's do this!

During socializing, your goal is to notice when your attention becomes self-focused or distracted by your surroundings and to redirect it to the task of socializing; that is, making conversation, maintaining eye contact, listening to what others are saying, asking questions, giving compliments and so on.

It might sound a little scary at first, especially if you're feeling anxious—and that's normal. With practice, you will get better. Do your best and keep trying again and again, as this builds your confidence. It's useful to reflect afterward and make notes in your journal. Notice how practicing influences the quality of social interactions over time.

When socializing, remember: people may look calm even when they don't feel calm, because often they have a lot on their minds—everyone has their own worries. People are not solely focused on finding flaws in you or judging you negatively. Or they're distracted by their phones! So, you're usually wrong when you think people can see that you're nervous. Like you, most people want connection and no one is entirely happy with how they come across or get on with others.

If conversations dry up, silence is OK. You don't have to take responsibility to keep a conversation going. Stay curious, put your focus outside: notice if other people are showing signs of anxiety. Believe that people won't think less of you or dislike you because you're anxious. Would you feel empathy for someone who was anxious? If the answer's yes, others probably feel the same. Afterward, avoid a postmortem of the situation as best as you can—try the *distracting thoughts* tips (page 52), or breathing exercises (page 74) instead.

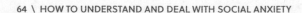

Confronting avoidance

It's really important to confront avoidance because avoidance is the most powerful way to strengthen social anxiety's grip on us. The more we avoid situations, the more we assume our negative thoughts are true. While avoidance may give us short-term relief from anxiety, we don't get the chance to test negative thoughts, disprove worst-case scenarios or experience positive connections, which sadly grows self-criticism and makes anxiety worse.

We must break this vicious cycle by approaching situations that make us anxious. Initially, this might elevate our anxiety, but science shows our fight-flight-freeze response will reach a plateau and then fall. The more we put ourselves in challenging situations over and over, the more anxiety will lessen. Your confidence to cope strengthens while self-criticism reduces and you'll actually enjoy interacting, which you totally deserve.

Write a list of your avoidance behaviors, like avoiding people, eye contact, talking or specific situations.

Confronting safety behaviors

Avoidance and safety behaviors often go hand-in-hand. We covered safety behaviors, which are a subtle form of avoidance, on page 29. If you want to deal with social anxiety, you will need to confront your safety behaviors. This might seem daunting at first, but with small, gradual steps, you can work up to facing your fears.

Safety behaviors can look like this: *Avoiding eye contact. Not speaking up. Letting others do the talking. Rehearsing what to say. Sticking to safe places or people. Gripping objects tightly. Avoiding talking about yourself. Keeping busy. Using a phone or earphones to avoid talking. Using alcohol or drugs.*

What do you do to prevent your worst-case scenario happening? How do you keep yourself safe from social embarrassment? What do you do to make sure you don't make mistakes? What do you do so people don't notice your anxiety?

Write a list of your safety behaviors.

Face your fears

You don't need special skills to change your behavior. But gradually doing things differently will release you from the social anxiety trap and leave you feeling comfortable being yourself.

Of course, behaving differently means facing our fears. This could mean speaking up more in groups, accepting invites or making more eye contact. Letting go of safety behaviors gives you permission to be yourself, to engage in situations and make connections instead of avoiding them. Although this might seem frightening, such behavioral experiments are a tried and tested way to overcome fears.

Fear is nothing more than an obstacle standing in the way of you making progress. In facing your fears, you can move forward with greater strength, resilience and wisdom. When trying new behaviors or facing uncomfortable situations, keep an open mind and stay curious about what happens.

What social fears might you be able to face?

You've got this!

Behavioral experiments require letting go of safety behaviors or approaching situations that are anxiety-provoking, which can feel risky and requires courage. You're doing amazingly by taking proactive steps. But you might worry, "What if the worst-case scenario happens?" Remember, the thing you most fear rarely happens, and if it does happen, you will cope. Also, it's unlikely to be as catastrophic as you imagined.

When trying new behaviors, take it slowly. Every small step is progress—keep going. Everyone has good and bad days, and mistakes are a part of the process. Celebrate your wins, big and small—you've got this.

Create an anxiety staircase

To test your fears, it's helpful to try some experiments that encourage a change in behavior and where you can challenge your anxiety.

Of course, this means coming out of your comfort zone. So, it's helpful to do this one step at a time, starting with social situations that create mild anxiety and then building up to more challenging ones as your coping skills and confidence grow. By the time you reach the toughest steps, they might not be so anxiety-triggering.

It's beneficial to order situations as a staircase you are about to climb with the least challenging step at the bottom and the most at the top, like in this diagram.

Create your own anxiety staircase. Consider these questions when doing so: How many people are there and who are they? Are they familiar? Is the place familiar? What am I doing? Where and when am I doing it?

Most anxious

Offer to lead a team meeting at work

Say more about myself and initiate meeting friends or colleagues for coffee

Socialize with new people other than close friends or family

Have lunch with coworkers and make conversation

Talk to people and stay, instead of finding excuses to leave or looking at phone

Say at least two things when in a group or meeting

Reply to a group message and offer my ideas

Least anxious

Please remember, there isn't a right or wrong order for your experiments. If you are OK to start with tougher steps, then go for it. The main thing is to start. Do it! You will feel so pleased with yourself.

Keep experimenting

Studies show that doing behavioral experiments regularly is more effective than random one-offs. Doing several every week has the most valuable results—consistency and perseverance are key. Keep track of your experiments by asking yourself these questions and record your progress in your journal!

Safety behaviors	Looking at my phone to hide, pretending I didn't hear when someone asks a question.
What is the worst-case scenario if you don't keep "safe"?	They will think I'm boring, I'll say the wrong thing and blush.
What will you do differently?	Stop hiding and stay present.
What happened? (Stick to facts.)	I blushed but a nice conversation flowed.
What does this mean?	People don't judge or care if I blush, I'm not boring. Experimenting is fun!

Dealing with physical symptoms

While anxiety can feel dreadful, it is hugely important to know that it's not dangerous or harmful and it can't physically hurt you. It's simply your thoughts spiralling out of control and triggering your fight-flight-freeze stress response. The good news is, it's entirely possible to learn how to deal with those horrible symptoms, such as your heart racing so rapidly it's ready to burst out of your chest, or the stomach-churning nausea.

Prolonged stress, however, can lead to autoimmune diseases, decreased immunity, heart disease, insomnia, obesity and respiratory infections. Thankfully, learning to regulate your emotional and physical response during high anxiety is do-able using techniques such as deep breathing, progressive muscle relaxation and mindfulness. Read on to find out how.

What physical symptoms would you like to deal with?

The importance of breathing

Breathing plays an important role in anxiety because it determines our physical state. When our body is triggered by threat into fight-flight-freeze, our breathing rate increases, making it harder for our bodies to keep the optimum balance between the oxygen we are breathing in and the carbon dioxide we are breathing out. If our bodies cannot return our carbon dioxide to ideal levels quickly enough, we are likely to feel dizzy or experience headaches, light-headedness, numbness and tingling or tense muscles.

Breathing techniques help by interrupting the sympathetic nervous system (which produces the fight-flight-freeze response) and triggering the parasympathetic nervous system instead, which calms the stress response, slows your breathing and lessens your anxiety levels.

With regular practice, preferably daily, breathing techniques help you cope better during a highly anxious situation. Plus, they are really relaxing!

Deep breathing

Deep breathing is a soothing and easy technique to learn to help regulate your breathing. Breathe the rainbow is a fun and effective exercise for anyone. Take slow deep breaths, hold for a few seconds, then breathe out while visualizing your favorite things to match each color. This exercise will help you to relax and clear your mind, reducing anxiety.

- Red—ripe apples, roses, strawberries
- Orange—sunset, sunrise, sweet mangoes
- Yellow—sun, sunflowers, daffodils
- Green—trees, grass, hills
- Blue—sky, sea, ocean
- Purple—ripe berries, grapes, pansies
- Pink—roses, tulips, other blossoms

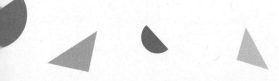

Progressive muscle relaxation

Many people tense up when they're feeling anxious. You might hold that tension in your jaw, your shoulders, or by taking shallow breaths. Anxiety has an effect on your body, physically, which is why it can feel awfully exhausting. But the good news is, you can actually reduce that tension using progressive muscle relaxation— where you purposefully clench your muscles then release them.

First, close your eyes and focus on your breathing for 2 minutes. Say out loud or in your mind (whichever feels comfortable) inhaling "calm," exhaling "tension."

- Face—scrunch your forehead like you're frowning, then relax. Clench your jaw, then relax. Notice the difference.
- Neck—roll your head slowly from side to side. Notice any tension.

- Shoulders—roll your shoulders back then forward. Shrug them up and down. Notice them relaxing.
- Arms—tense your biceps for 5 seconds then release. Clench your hands in a fist and release.
- Stomach—tense your muscles tightly then relax. Notice your chest rising and falling when breathing.
- Legs—tense your calf muscles tightly then relax.
- Feet—point your toes up for 5 seconds then wriggle them to release tension.

Keep practicing this as often as you can. Once you're familiar with the technique, this brilliant tool can be used on the go anywhere and everywhere. Imagine feeling super confident before a presentation because you're able to instantly relax and feel in control.

Mindful breathing

Science shows that mindfulness calms our stress response, untangling us from anxiety while creating a sense of physical and emotional nourishment. By not getting caught up in our thoughts about the past or future, it helps us remain calm and in control.

Try this 3-minute exercise.

Sitting comfortably, close your eyes and take deep breaths. Place your feet flat on the floor. Notice your soles where they touch the ground. Now, place a hand on your stomach. Take three deep breaths and focus your attention on your breathing. Notice your stomach rising and falling with each in-breath and out-breath. If your mind wanders that's OK, gently guide it back to your breathing. Now, breathe in for a count of five, then hold your breath for a count of five, and breathe out slowly for a count of five, for 3 minutes. When ready, open your eyes. How are you feeling?

Quick anxiety calmers

When you need to calm your anxiety, breathing techniques are natural tranquilizers for the nervous system. Use them before, during or after social situations to help regulate physical symptoms and emotions, and to pause those negative thoughts.

These simple and brilliantly effective little exercises ground you instantly into the moment.

Hand breathing meditation

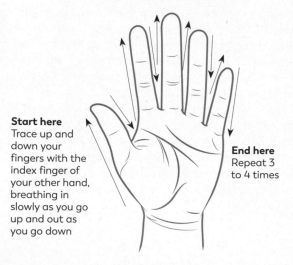

Start here
Trace up and down your fingers with the index finger of your other hand, breathing in slowly as you go up and out as you go down

End here
Repeat 3 to 4 times